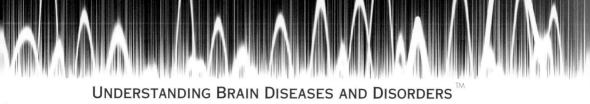

UNDERSTANDING BRAIN DISEASES AND DISORDERS™

BRAIN TUMORS

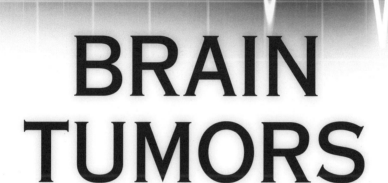

LOUIS J. COOK
AND
JERI FREEDMAN

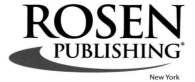

ROSEN
PUBLISHING®

New York

Published in 2012 by The Rosen Publishing Group, Inc.
29 East 21st Street, New York, NY 10010

Copyright © 2012 by The Rosen Publishing Group, Inc.

First Edition

Library of Congress Cataloging-in-Publication Data

Cook, Louis J.
Brain tumors/Louis J. Cook, Jeri Freedman—1st ed.
     p. cm.—(Understanding brain diseases and disorders)
Includes bibliographical references and index.
ISBN 978-1-4488-5544-5 (library binding)
1. Brain—Tumors—Juvenile literature.
2. Brain—Tumors—Treatment—Juvenile literature. I. Freedman, Jeri. II. Title.
RC280.B7.C66 2012
616.99'481—dc23

                                                                    2011022613

Manufactured in China

CPSIA Compliance Information: Batch #W12YA: For further information, contact Rosen Publishing, New York, New York, at 1-800-237-9932.

CONTENTS

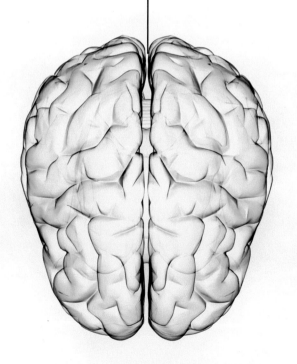

Introduction

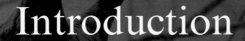

The brain is a complex organ, which controls our basic body functions, senses, thoughts, feelings, memories, speech, movement, and more. The spinal cord and nerves carry messages between the brain and the rest of the organs in the body. This entire communication system is known as the central nervous system (CNS).

Brain tumors are masses of unnecessary cells that can grow in the brain and affect its functioning. Scientists believe that most brain tumors are the result of genetic mutations, or changes in the genes, that normally keep cells from reproducing in an uncontrolled manner.

The brain and spinal cord have many kinds of cells, which can result in the development of a variety of tumors. Some types of brain tumors are seen more often in adults, while others are seen more frequently in children. Most occur equally in men and women, but some are more common in one gender than the other. Depending on the type of tumor and its location, each may have a different outlook and treatment.

A brain tumor can be either malignant (cancerous) or benign (noncancerous), but in either case it can threaten a person's health and life. A brain tumor can compress normal brain tissue within the confined area of the skull; as a result, the brain tissue can be damaged or destroyed.

Unfortunately, brain tumors are not extremely rare. According to the National Brain Tumor Society, in the United States approximately nineteen out of every one hundred thousand people develop brain and central nervous system tumors every year. Brain cancer is the most common type of cancer that causes death in people under the age of thirty-five.

Because brain tumors are not associated with lifestyle or environmental factors that most people encounter, there is no known way to guard against them at this time. But new research and treatments offer great hope for a breakthrough and a possible cure for this dreaded disease.

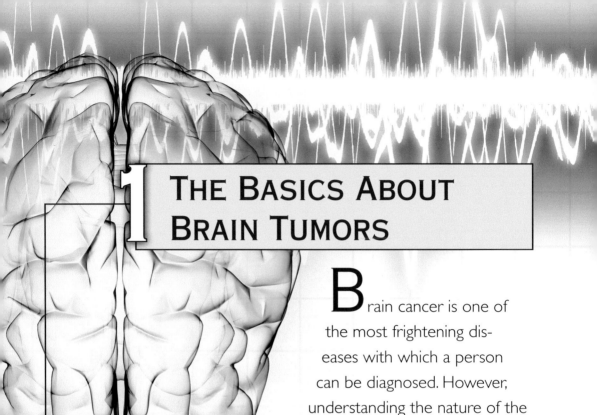

1 THE BASICS ABOUT BRAIN TUMORS

Brain cancer is one of the most frightening diseases with which a person can be diagnosed. However, understanding the nature of the disease can help a person begin to cope. To understand why brain tumors pose so much danger, we will first examine the different parts of the brain and their normal functions. We will then take a look at the different kinds of tumors that can affect the brain and spinal cord.

Understanding the Brain

The brain and the spinal cord together make up the central nervous system (CNS), which sends signals to and receives them from all parts of the body. Different sections of the brain control various physical and mental functions.

The biggest area of the brain is the cerebrum. It consists of two halves, or hemispheres, connected by a series of nerves. The left hemisphere of the brain controls the right side of the body, and the right hemisphere of the brain controls the left side of the body. Each hemisphere is further divided into four sections called lobes.

- **Frontal lobes:** Located at the front of the brain, they control reasoning, judgment, inhibition, mood, attention, some body movement, and the bowel and bladder. Damage to the frontal lobes can affect one's sense of consequences and notions of right and wrong, resulting in reckless or rule-breaking behavior.
- **Temporal lobes:** Located in the lower part of the cerebrum, they control hearing-related activity and long-term memory. In most people, the left temporal lobe is responsible for understanding language. In about 5 percent of people, the language function is located in the right temporal lobe.
- **Parietal lobes:** Located in the upper center of the cerebrum, they process sensory information and spatial orientation. They also play a role in reading, writing, and performing mathematical calculations.
- **Occipital lobes:** Located at the back of the cerebrum, they control vision. The right occipital lobe processes information from the left eye, while the left occipital lobe processes information from the right eye.

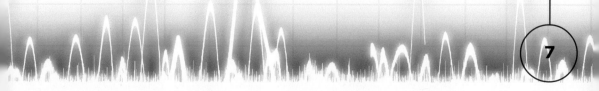

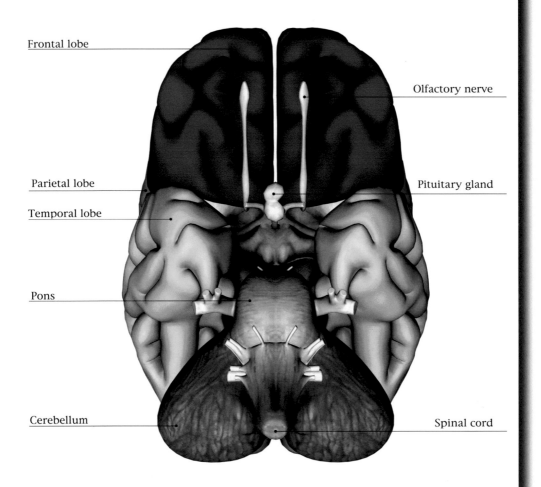

Frontal lobe

Olfactory nerve

Parietal lobe

Pituitary gland

Temporal lobe

Pons

Cerebellum

Spinal cord

This underside view of the brain shows the cerebellum (shown here in pink), part of the brain stem, and most of the major lobes of the cerebrum. Each part of the brain plays a different role in our body functions, sensations, emotions, thoughts, and behaviors.

Below the cerebrum is the brain stem, which is divided into three parts: the midbrain, which is closest to the cerebrum; the pons; and the medulla oblongata. Information related to sight, hearing, smell, movement, and balance is transmitted from nerves through the spinal cord to the brain stem via twelve cranial nerves. The areas that control sleeping and waking and involuntary body functions—those we don't control consciously, such as the beating of the heart—are also located in the brain stem. The brain contains two main types of cells: nerve cells, which send and receive electrical signals; and glial cells, which provide the supporting and protective structure for nerve cells.

What Are Brain Tumors?

In cancer, a group of normal or abnormal cells reproduces and grows out of control, forming a mass, or tumor. When a brain tumor occurs, the ever-growing mass of unnecessary cells compresses and damages other cells in the brain, interfering with brain function. The tumor pushes brain tissue around, creates pressure by pressing against the bones of the skull, and infiltrates (or invades) healthy brain tissue and the areas around the nerves. As a result, the tumor damages the tissues in the brain.

Depending on where a brain tumor is located, it will affect different aspects of movement, senses, and behavior. There are a

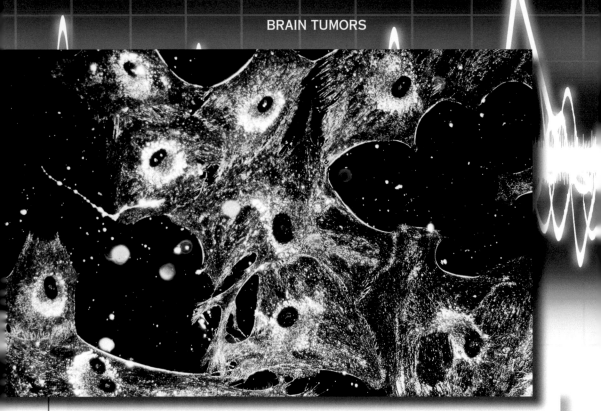

These cancer cells, magnified under a microscope, were grown from a human brain tumor. Cancer cells grow and divide uncontrollably, forming new, abnormal cells that can invade healthy tissue.

large variety of brain tumors that grow from different types of cells. In all, there are more than 120 types of brain tumors. Since there are so many different kinds of brain tumors, it can be helpful to understand how doctors describe and classify them.

Primary and Metastatic Brain Tumors

Brain cancer is divided into two categories: primary brain cancer and metastatic brain cancer. Primary brain cancer results from an abnormal growth of cells that starts in the brain itself. According to the National Cancer Institute, each year in the

United States more than 35,000 people are told they have a tumor that started in the brain.

Secondary brain cancer, also called metastatic brain cancer, comes from cancer that starts in another body organ, such as the breast, lung, colon, or liver. The cancer metastasizes, or spreads, from the original site to other areas of the body, such as the brain. Cancerous cells from another part of the body travel through the blood to the brain. Once there, the cells start reproducing in the same out-of-control way as the cells in the original tumor. Once cancer has metastasized, the patient has a lesser chance of survival than if the cancer is caught before it spreads.

Metastatic brain tumors are the most common type of brain tumor. According to the American Brain Tumor Association (ABTA), the number of cases of metastatic brain tumors diagnosed each year is at least four times greater than that of primary brain tumors.

Benign and Malignant Brain Tumors

There are two types of primary brain tumors: benign and malignant. A benign tumor is a cluster of cells that builds up in the brain. It usually grows slowly and does not invade nearby tissue or spread to other parts of the body. Such a tumor may present serious problems if it affects nearby brain tissue, causing symptoms such as loss of sight or hearing. It may become life threatening if it affects critical structures in the brain, such as major blood vessels.

Malignant tumors grow quickly and aggressively invade nearby tissue. Malignant tumors are always life threatening because there is a high likelihood that they will invade and damage tissue in the brain. Although no one knows why, some benign tumors, if left untreated for a long period of time, will change into malignant tumors.

Primary brain tumors that are malignant can spread from the brain to the spinal cord. However, unlike many other forms of cancer, it is rare for tumors that start in the brain to metastasize and spread to other parts of the body.

Types of Primary Brain Tumors

Primary brain tumors are divided into two main groups: glial tumors and nonglial tumors. Glial tumors, also known as gliomas, grow from cells in the fibers supporting the nerve cells in the brain. Nonglial tumors grow from the nerves, glands, or blood vessels in the brain.

Glial Tumors or Gliomas

The most common type of glial tumor is called an astrocytoma. This type of tumor grows from glial cells that are called astrocytes because they are star-shaped (*astro* is Latin for "star," and *cyto* means "cell"). This type of tumor can occur in almost any part of the brain. In children, this type of tumor usually grows slowly, but in adults, it can be very aggressive. The fastest-growing kind of astrocytoma is known as a glioblastoma. It is the most common malignant brain tumor in adults.

The axons of nerve cells in the central nervous system have an insulating sheath made up of a fatty material called myelin. This substance helps nerve cells send signals to one another. Brain cells called oligodendrocytes create myelin. A tumor starting in these cells is called an oligodendroglioma. This type of tumor primarily

This CT scan of a patient's brain shows a large glioblastoma (shown here in orange-red). A glioblastoma is the most invasive and fastest-growing type of glial tumor.

affects young to middle-aged adults. Oligodendrogliomas can grow into nearby brain tissue, where they cannot be completely removed by surgery.

Another type of glioma is the ependymoma. The brain has ventricles, which are butterfly-shaped openings in the center of the brain through which spinal fluid flows around the central nervous system. Ependymomas grow from the cells that line these ventricles and the spinal cord. According to the

University of Maryland Greenebaum Cancer Center, about 10 percent of brain tumors in children are ependymomas.

Nonglial Tumors

One type of nonglial tumor is the chordoma. Chordomas usually occur in adults in their twenties and thirties. They are slow-growing tumors that can metastasize. Chordomas grow from leftover bits of the pre-spinal-cord structure that is replaced by the spinal cord as a fetus develops.

Medulloblastoma is an aggressive, malignant tumor that occurs most commonly in the cerebellum, the part of the brain above and behind the brain stem, at the back of the head. Although this type of tumor sometimes appears in adults, it is more common in children. According to St. Jude Children's Research Hospital, about 20 percent of childhood brain tumors are medulloblastomas. They are slightly more common in boys than in girls.

Lymphoma is a type of cancer that grows from the white blood cells (lymphocytes). These immune system cells travel through the body fighting infection. Lymphoma can occur in many different parts of the body. When it begins in the central nervous system (the brain and spinal cord), it is called primary central nervous system (CNS) lymphoma. In this form of cancer, the lymphocytes grow out of control, forming tumors in the brain and sometimes in the spinal cord as well.

False Brain Tumors

In Latin, the name of the condition known as pseudotumor cerebri literally means "false brain tumor," and that is exactly what it is. It is not a tumor at all, but a buildup of fluid in the brain. The fluid buildup creates increased pressure within the skull. This process results in symptoms typically associated with brain tumors, including head-aches, dizziness, nausea, and double vision. A complication that can occur with this condition is partial or permanent loss of vision.

To treat pseudotumor cerebri, doctors often prescribe drugs to help drain excess fluid from the brain. Another possible treat-ment includes lumbar puncture, or spinal tap, to relieve pressure in the brain and prevent vision problems. If necessary, a patient can undergo surgery to relieve pressure on the optic nerve.

Benign Nonglial Tumors

Several types of nonglial tumors are benign. Though not malig-nant or life threatening, they can cause serious health prob-lems. Tumors found in the central nervous system are among the few benign tumors that require aggressive treatment and removal because of the sensitivity of their location. Benign tumors can place pressure on sensitive nerve and brain tis-sues, and they can harm the normal functioning of the ner-vous system.

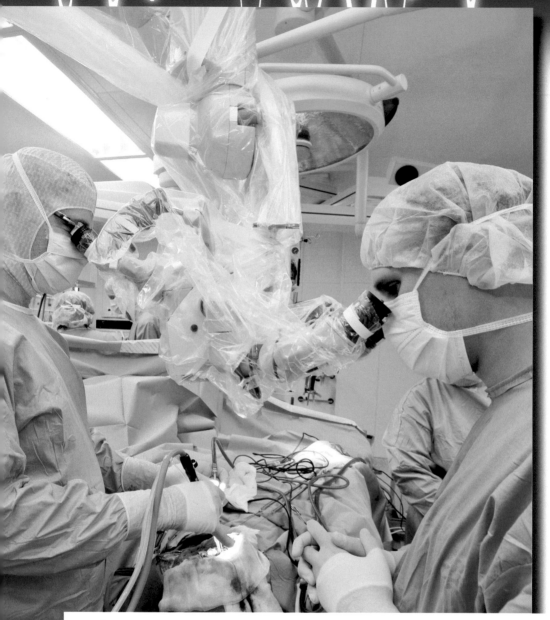

Neurosurgeons look through a surgical microscope as they work to remove a patient's benign brain tumor. Though noncancerous, benign brain tumors can press on the normal brain structures inside the skull.

For example, a meningioma is a tumor that originates in the meninges, the layers of tissue that make up the outer covering of the brain and spinal cord. According to the ABTA, about 27 percent of all primary brain tumors are meningiomas, making them the most common brain tumor in adults. Some meningiomas grow near the optic nerve, squeezing it and causing vision loss.

According to the Stanford University School of Medicine, about 10 percent of brain tumors grow from cells of the pituitary gland. This gland in the brain releases hormones, or substances that regulate growth and body functions. One type of pituitary tumor is a pituitary adenoma, which is usually benign. It is rare in children and occurs primarily in adolescents and adults.

The pituitary gland is found inside the skull, just above the nasal passages. It is considered the master control gland of hormone production because it regulates the activity of most other glands in the body. It has a particularly important role in adolescence: it regulates the hormones that begin to be produced at the onset of puberty, triggering all of the physical changes that usher teens into adulthood.

Pituitary adenomas usually do not spread beyond the area of the pituitary. Though benign, they can cause serious health problems. Because the space is so tight in that part of the skull, even a small growth can create crowding and constrict pituitary tissue. This can result in vision problems and hormone deficiencies. Larger adenomas, called macroadenomas, can even release their own pituitary hormones. This can result in hormone overproduction and related growth, metabolism, menstruation, ovulation, and sperm-production problems.

A benign tumor found deep inside the brain is especially dangerous because surgery to remove it may damage vital brain centers. In such cases, radiation may be used to shrink the tumor. A benign tumor located closer to the brain's surface can usually be removed surgically with minimal risk and complications.

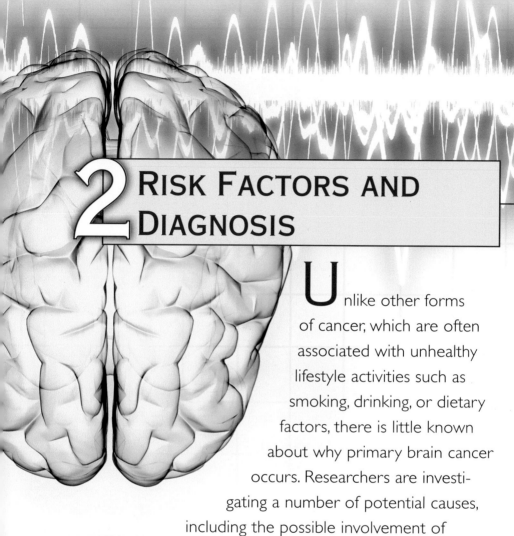

2 RISK FACTORS AND DIAGNOSIS

Unlike other forms of cancer, which are often associated with unhealthy lifestyle activities such as smoking, drinking, or dietary factors, there is little known about why primary brain cancer occurs. Researchers are investigating a number of potential causes, including the possible involvement of viruses, chemicals, and genetic factors.

Possible Causes

Most brain cancer is the result of genetic mutations (changes) in the genes that normally keep cells from reproducing in an uncontrolled manner. These genes are called tumor suppressor genes. When one of these genes is altered or deleted, the brake on cell growth is removed, and tumors can form.

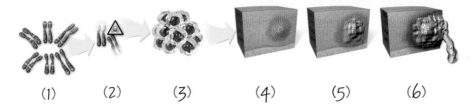

(1)   (2)   (3)   (4)   (5)   (6)

Malignant tumors are caused by changes in the genes carried in the chromosomes (1) in human cells. Damage to the genes and chromosomes (2) can cause cancerous cells to multiply (3) and then form a tumor within tissue (4–6).

Scientists believe some forms of brain cancer are inherited. However, brain tumors also occur in people with no family history of such tumors. Brain cancer may be the result of spontaneous mutation in the genetic material carried in the egg or sperm cells, or from factors that researchers have not yet identified.

Brain cancer is associated with one environmental factor: exposure to vinyl chloride, a chemical used in making plastics. If one lives near a plant that uses vinyl chloride or a toxic waste site where this material may have been disposed of, then there is a chance that the chemical may have leaked into the local water supply. However, in most cases of brain tumors, there has not been exposure to this chemical.

Since brain cancer is not associated with specific lifestyle choices (such as cigarette smoking or alcohol consumption), there is no known way to guard against it at this time.

Symptoms of Brain Tumors

Brain cancer diagnosis starts with a discussion between the patient and a doctor about the symptoms the patient is experiencing. If the symptoms indicate the possibility of a brain tumor, then the patient will be given a neurological examination and possibly a brain scan. In some cases, a biopsy is performed.

Since different parts of the brain control different body functions and behaviors, brain tumors can produce many different types of symptoms. Symptoms depend on the kind of brain cancer a person has and the location of the tumor(s). Some symptoms may be specific to certain functions. For example, there may be effects on a person's sight, hearing, or balance. Other symptoms are more general. Symptoms commonly experienced by people suffering from brain tumors include:

- **Headaches:** Many people with a brain tumor experience headaches, which may last from several minutes to hours. The headaches may become worse if the person alters his or her position or coughs. However, headaches can have many causes, so this alone is not enough to indicate a brain tumor.
- **Vomiting:** Pressure inside the skull can result in nausea and vomiting, sometimes along with a headache.
- **Vision or hearing difficulties:** Vision and hearing problems can result from three causes: (1) Increased pressure in the skull can cause swelling of the optic nerve, leading to

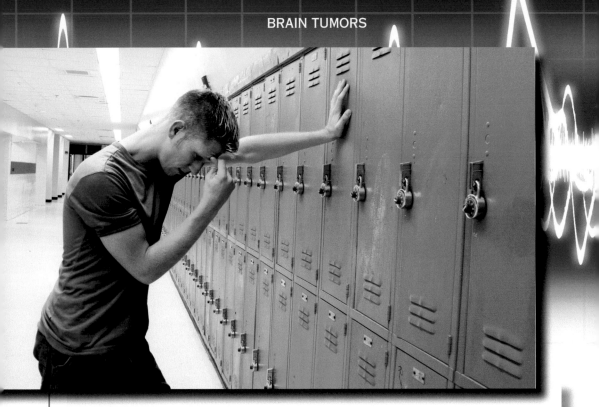

Severe headaches are one symptom of a brain tumor. Other symptoms include loss of balance; changes in one's ability to see, hear, or talk; and numbness, tingling, or weakness in the limbs.

double or blurred vision or partial loss of vision. (2) Tumors can grow in the occipital lobe region, where visual information is processed, resulting in apparent vision loss. (3) Tumors growing around or from sensory nerves can result in abnormal eye movement, crossed eyes, loss of vision, loss of hearing, or hearing strange sounds, such as ringing or buzzing.

- **Movement problems:** Sometimes, tumors affect areas of the brain that control movement. In that case, a person may have problems with weakness or paralysis and may experience difficulty with walking and coordination. If an area that controls balance is affected, a person may experience dizziness and/or have trouble maintaining balance.

- **Emotional or behavioral problems:** When a tumor is located in the parts of the brain that control reasoning, judgment, impulse control, communication, or emotion, the person may experience changes in behavior and emotional response. For example, an ordinarily quiet person may suddenly seem angry and aggressive. A normally controlled person may suddenly become extremely impulsive. Or, a typically intelligent and articulate person may suddenly develop problems in understanding or communicating. When the area of the brain responsible for memory is affected, a person will experience memory problems.
- **Seizures:** Nerve cells communicate by sending and receiving electrical signals. When the electrical activity in the brain becomes disordered, as sometimes occurs with a brain tumor, it is called a seizure. Seizures result in a variety of symptoms ranging from unconsciousness to convulsions (involuntary muscle contractions that cause violent body movements).

Physical Examination

In a physical examination for a possible brain tumor or other neurological problem, the doctor tests the patient's reflexes, strength, muscle control, balance, and other physical factors.

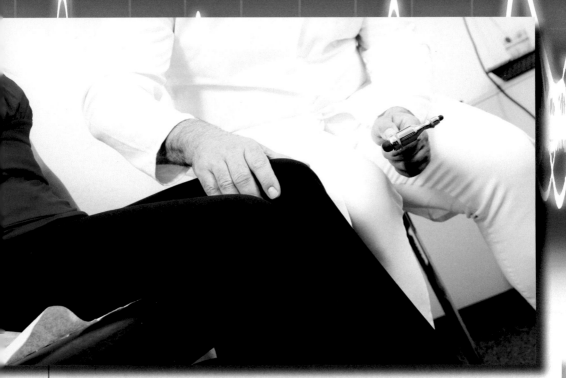

To detect the signs of a brain tumor, a doctor conducts an exam that measures the functioning of the nervous system. Testing the patient's reflexes is a common step.

The doctor may ask the patient to perform various physical actions to evaluate strength, muscle control, and coordination. He or she may test the patient's reflexes by tapping joints such as the knees with a tiny hammer. Sensory testing may also be conducted by touching parts of the arms or legs with a device that produces a pricking sensation. The doctor also tests the patient's mental responses.

If the physical and/or mental responses are not within the normal range, the doctor may order a brain scan or refer the patient to a doctor who specializes in treating diseases of the central nervous system. There are two types of specialists who treat diseases of the central nervous system. Neurologists treat diseases of the brain and spinal cord. Neurosurgeons perform surgery on the brain and spinal cord.

Imaging Tests

There are several different types of brain scans that are used to produce pictures of the brain. Brain scans use computer technology to create these pictures. They allow doctors to see all of the structures in the brain, including any abnormal ones. There are three main types of scans: magnetic resonance imaging (MRI), computed tomography (CT), and positron emission tomography (PET).

Magnetic Resonance Imaging (MRI) Scans

In an MRI scan, the patient is placed in a tubelike chamber. Inside the machine, large electromagnets surround the platform on which the patient lies. When they are turned on, the electromagnets create a magnetic field that interacts with the patient's tissue. This produces data that the computer can analyze to produce a detailed picture of the inside of the body part being imaged—in this case, the brain. Because MRIs do not use X-ray technology, they do not expose the patient to radiation. However, because they use magnetic fields, they can interact with pacemakers and metal implants, such as pins or plates used

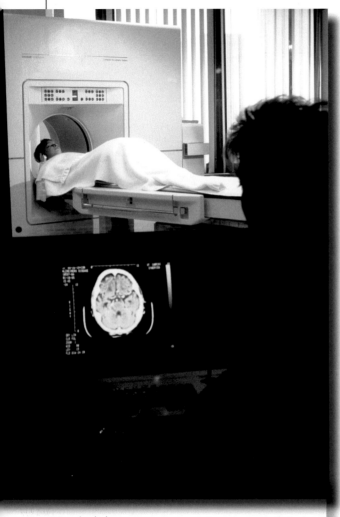

An MRI technician reads a patient's brain scan. An MRI is the most commonly used scan for detecting a brain tumor.

to repair broken bones. So, you should tell the doctor or imaging technician if you have any of these. MRIs take a series of pictures, each of which is a thin slice of the brain. The computer then combines all of the sequential pictures to produce a three-dimensional image of the brain.

Computed Tomography (CT) Scans

CT scans use X-ray technology and computer analysis to provide pictures of tissues, blood vessels, and bones. In order to make tissues stand out, a dye is often injected into the patient. Since this dye may contain iodine, people allergic to iodine should let the doctor or imaging technician know. CT scans can show bleeding and swelling, as well as some tumors.

Getting Support

Dealing with the diagnosis of, treatment of, and recovery from brain tumors can be a scary and stressful experience. For this reason, you may want to talk with a counselor who works with cancer patients and their families. In addition, there are a variety of support groups for people who are diagnosed with brain cancer and are undergoing cancer treatment. A list of such groups can be found on the Web sites of reputable organizations such as the American Cancer Society (http://www.cancer.org) and the National Brain Tumor Society (http://www.braintumor.org), as well as through recommendations at the facility where you obtain cancer treatment.

Positron Emission Tomography (PET) Scans

PET scans don't take a picture of the brain itself. Instead, they record activity in the different parts of the brain. The brain uses glucose, a type of sugar, as fuel. The PET scan helps doctors determine the activity in a tumor by showing how much glucose it is absorbing. To do the scan, a type of glucose is combined with a weak radioactive marker and injected into a patient. As the brain absorbs the glucose, the PET scan records the amount of radioactivity in specific areas, and this information is analyzed by a computer. PET scans are useful not only for identifying areas that contain tumor cells but also for locating scar tissue and brain tissue that has been destroyed by treatment.

27

Brain Tumor Biopsy

In a biopsy, a small piece of tissue is removed from a tumor. This tissue is examined in a laboratory to gain information about the structure of the cells in the tumor. In most cases of suspected brain cancer, when a biopsy is performed, a piece of bone is removed from the skull. A neurosurgeon then removes all or part of the tumor, and the bone is usually put back.

When a tumor is located in an area that is difficult to reach, the doctor may instead perform a closed biopsy. In this case, the surgeon drills a small hole in the skull, inserts a hollow needle into the tumor, and removes a piece of the tissue. The tissue is examined under a microscope to evaluate the tumor cells and grade the tumor.

Tumor Grading

Doctors give tumors grades to indicate how advanced the patient's cancer is. Tumor grading involves describing the characteristics or changes seen in cells as cancer progresses.

A widely accepted system for grading tumors is the one established by the World Health Organization (WHO). A tumor is assigned a grade based on how similar the cell structure is to that of normal cells, how fast the cells are growing, and how likely they are to spread. The higher the grade, the more advanced the tumor is.

```
5/ 3/83
SCAN 2    SLC 3

   83 MM
```

```
MG
GLU

19.4
18.3
17.2
16.2
15.1
14.0
13.0
11.9
10.8
 9.7
 8.6
 7.6
 6.5
 5.4
 4.3
 3.3
 2.2
 1.1
 0.1
```

This PET scan shows the brain of a man with a grade III astro-cytoma. The bright colors indicate an increased rate of glucose absorption in the area of the tumor.

For example, tumors that are self-contained (have not grown into surrounding tissue) and slow-growing are often called grade I. Such tumors are considered benign or mildly malignant. Malignant tumors, which have grown into surrounding tissue, are categorized as grade II, III, or IV, according to how advanced they are. Sometimes, such tumors are also referred to using the terms "low grade," "mid-grade," and "high grade," depending on their severity.

MYTHS AND FACTS

Myth: Using a cell phone can cause brain tumors.

Fact: So far, controlled studies have not shown a relation-
ship between brain cancer and cell phone use. Some
people are concerned about cell phones because they
emit radiofrequency (RF) energy, a form of electromagnetic radiation, and they are used close to the head.
Electromagnetic radiation can be divided into two
types: ionizing (high-frequency) and non-ionizing (low-
frequency) radiation. Exposure to ionizing radiation, such
as the radiation produced by X-ray machines, can raise
one's cancer risk. However, according to the National
Cancer Institute, there is currently no conclusive evidence
that the low-frequency radiation emitted by cell phones
raises cancer risk.

Myth: Keeping an upbeat attitude, meditating, watching funny
movies, or praying will cure brain cancer.

Fact: Only proper medical treatment will cure brain and
other forms of cancer. However, there is some evidence
that people with a good mental attitude recover better
and cope better with their illness. This may be because

these approaches reduce stress, which adversely affects the body. Also, such people are more hopeful and confident, which may lead them to be more active in attempting to improve their condition. It is important to emphasize, though, that cancer cannot be cured by any mental or spiritual approach alone. Medical treatment is still necessary.

Myth: Alternative or holistic health techniques can cure cancer.
Fact: Alternative health techniques, such as acupuncture, massage, or herbal supplements, can help treat some symptoms resulting from cancer treatment, like pain, nausea, or emotional stress. By themselves, however, these alternative techniques will not make a tumor go away. Conventional treatment is still required.

After a biopsy sample is taken, a pathologist (a doctor who specializes in analyzing diseases) examines the tissue under a microscope and indicates whether the tumor is benign or malignant, what type of cells are involved in the tumor, and what the grade of the tumor is. This analysis provides the doctor with information that will help in establishing the most appropriate treatment.

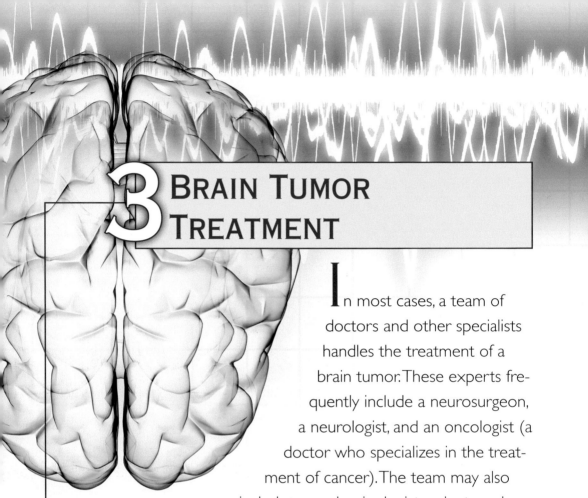

3 BRAIN TUMOR TREATMENT

In most cases, a team of doctors and other specialists handles the treatment of a brain tumor. These experts frequently include a neurosurgeon, a neurologist, and an oncologist (a doctor who specializes in the treatment of cancer). The team may also include an endocrinologist, a doctor who treats diseases in the hormone-secreting glands. Physicians treat tumors with one or more of the following techniques: surgery, chemotherapy, and radiation. Scientists are also researching and testing newer and more advanced techniques for treating tumors.

Surgery for Brain Tumors

Surgery is the primary technique used to treat tumors whenever it is possible. Surgery performed on the brain is called craniotomy.

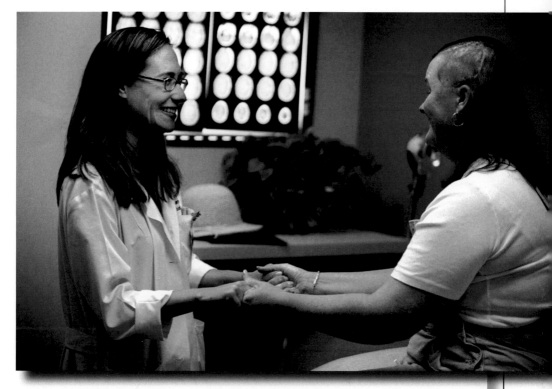

Neurosurgeon Edie Zusman greets her patient, Roberta Stead, who is recovering well a week after surgery to remove a brain tumor.

Prior to surgery, a patient may be given medications, such as steroids, to reduce swelling and inflammation. The neurosurgeon will attempt to remove the tumor in a process called resectioning. The goal is to remove the tumor while causing minimal disturbance to the surrounding structures.

A common surgical technique used in removing tumors is microsurgery. In this type of surgery, the surgeon looks through a mounted high-powered microscope. The microscope makes the tumor and surrounding tissue look much larger than they would with the naked eye. As a result, it is easier for the surgeon to separate the tumor from the surrounding tissue and remove it. The surgeon tries to remove the entire tumor, if possible. If it is not completely removed, the tumor could grow back.

Sometimes, because of its location, it is not possible to remove the entire tumor without causing significant damage to the surrounding tissue. In this case, the surgeon removes as much of the tumor as possible in order to reduce the symptoms it is causing. Then, the patient is treated with chemotherapy and/or radiation in an attempt to destroy any cancer cells in the remaining section of tumor.

Radiation Therapy

In radiation therapy, high-energy X-rays or other types of radiation are applied to a tumor to destroy the cancer cells. Doctors often use this approach when a tumor is located in a place that makes surgery impossible, or when a tumor can only be partially removed.

Radiation therapy can be external or internal. In internal radiation therapy, pellets of radioactive material are implanted directly into the tumor, where the radiation will kill the surrounding cells. Internal radiation therapy is most often used for tumors that are small and hard to remove.

When radiation is applied externally, a machine is used to focus a high-energy X-ray beam on the area to be treated. In conventional radiation therapy, a patient receives a number of treatments, using small amounts of radiation, over a series of weeks. When the tumor is located in one specific area of the brain, focused radiation treatments are used. In this case, a machine delivers a focused energy beam directly to the specific site of the tumor.

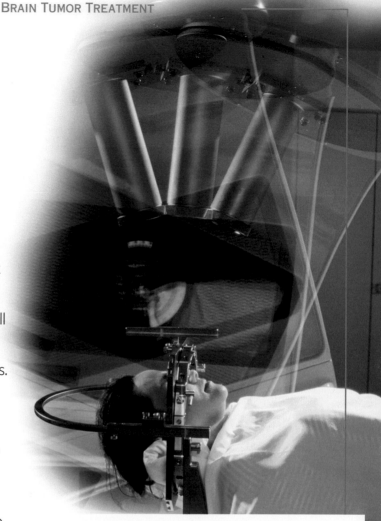

A patient undergoes stereotactic radiosurgery at UCLA Medical Center. The treatment uses a highly focused beam of radiation to target the cancer cells.

If a patient has multiple tumors or metastasized tumors, then another type of radiation therapy, called whole brain radiation therapy (WBRT), is used. In this case, a wide beam of radiation is focused on the entire brain.

An alternative to conventional external radiation therapy is stereotactic radiosurgery (SRS). It cannot be used in all cases, but if the size and location of the tumor are appropriate, this technique is the preferred one. First, an MRI or CT scan is used to create a three-dimensional map of the area where the tumor is located. This information allows a computer to precisely establish the location of the tumor. Doctors can use this technique to treat a tumor with a single high dose of radiation in one session, rather than multiple smaller doses over many weeks. If appropriate, a machine can be used to deliver a beam of radiation to the exact site of the tumor, often from multiple directions. Stereotactic imaging can also be used to place radioactive pellets that will kill tumors with internal radiation therapy.

Short-term side effects of radiation therapy occur immediately after treatment. They include tiredness, nausea, loss of appetite, hair loss in the area being irradiated, and short-term memory loss. In most cases, the majority of these symptoms improve once the treatments are finished.

Sometimes, after they have been killed, the dead tumor cells reform and become a new mass in the brain. Such a mass can cause the same type of symptoms as a tumor—memory loss, headaches, and personality or behavioral changes. The new mass may also look like a tumor on a brain scan. Such masses are usually surgically removed or treated with steroids.

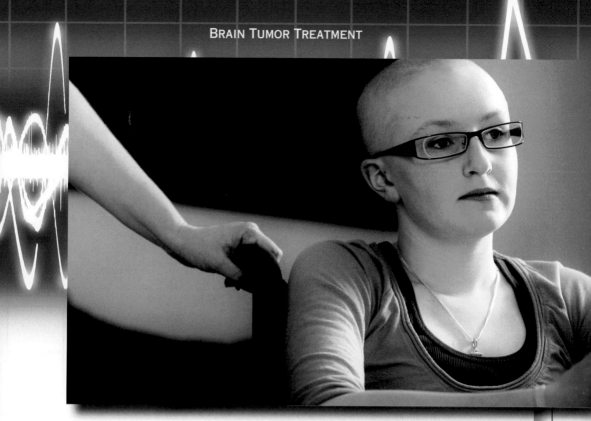

Hair loss occurs when chemotherapy drugs damage the quickly dividing cells of the hair follicles along with cancerous cells.

Chemotherapy

Conventional chemotherapy consists of a combination of medications that are taken orally or infused intravenously (directly into a vein). These medications kill fast-growing and dividing cells. Since cancer cells are constantly growing and dividing, the drugs help halt their rapid and uncontrolled growth. However, the medications may also affect other normally growing and dividing cells in the body, such as hair cells. This is why it is common for patients to lose their hair during chemotherapy.

Because the chemicals used in chemotherapy are so strong, they are usually given in a series of treatments at intervals. This allows the patient to rest and recover from the harsh effects of chemotherapy between treatments. Side effects of chemotherapy include hair loss, tiredness, chills, shortness of breath, nausea, and tingling in the patient's limbs.

After treatment, it is important for patients to continue to see their doctors regularly to make sure that the tumor does not recur. When a tumor has been treated successfully and the cancer cells stop multiplying, the patient is said to be in remission. There is no way to tell if the tumor will or will not recur after entering remission, so it is important to continue to see the doctor periodically. Most likely, a brain scan will be used to make sure that the tumor is not recurring.

Future Treatments for Brain Tumors

Doctors are interested in developing new ways to treat brain tumors that are less invasive, are more effective, and produce fewer side effects. The following are some new approaches being explored in cancer treatment.

Improved Chemotherapy and Radiation Therapy

As mentioned earlier, chemotherapy drugs have unpleasant side effects, including hair loss, tiredness, chills, shortness of breath, and nausea. Therefore, finding better chemotherapy drugs is a major area of research.

Today, the most commonly used chemotherapy drugs for treating brain cancer are carmustine, often referred to with the initials BCNU, and lomustine, often called CCNU. However, there are dozens of new combinations of chemicals being tested in the hope of developing better chemotherapy agents.

One approach to finding new chemotherapy drugs focuses on developing drugs that would affect only the type of cell that composes the tumor. This would result in fewer side effects from the killing of other healthy

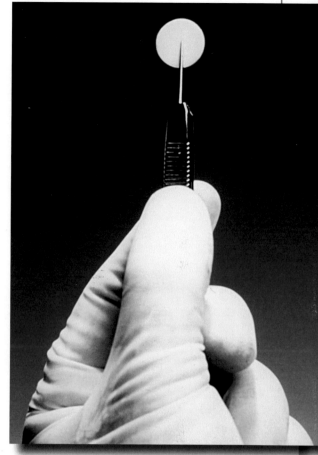

This dissolvable wafer, which can be implanted during surgery, contains the chemotherapy drug carmustine (BCNU). The wafer releases the drug at the tumor site.

cells during cancer treatment. Another approach is combining chemotherapy agents with other compounds to aid in their delivery. For instance, drugs are being combined with artificially produced forms of fat molecules (liposomes) to better penetrate the tumor cells. Cancer drugs that piggyback on liposomes are more effective because they are delivered into the heart of the tumor. This approach is called liposomal therapy.

In treating brain tumors, doctors face an obstacle that they don't have to deal with when treating other types of cancer. This obstacle is the blood-brain barrier. It consists of an interlacing series of blood vessels and cells that filter blood entering the brain. The blood-brain barrier removes potentially damaging substances from the blood before they can reach and affect the brain. Unfortunately, it also blocks many chemotherapy drugs that could help treat brain cancer. Researchers are working to find drugs that would make this barrier permeable to chemotherapy agents that cannot presently cross it.

One new approach to chemotherapy uses polymer wafer implants. In this approach, wafers made of a biodegradable material are saturated with a chemotherapy drug. When a tumor is removed, the wafers are inserted into the hole. They slowly dissolve, delivering the chemotherapy agent directly to the tumor site to kill any remaining cancer cells. This approach can be used to deliver a higher dose of chemotherapy medication than is possible with conventional intravenous or oral approaches because there is less need to worry about the drug's effects on normal cells.

Research is also being undertaken to find medications that patients can take to protect themselves from the side effects of

Using Heat to Treat Tumors

Some researchers are testing a variety of approaches that use heat in order to boost the power of cancer drugs and kill cancer cells without harming healthy cells. According to an article from ScienceDaily.com, bioengineers at Duke University have been working to design a thin catheter that can fit into the large blood vessels of the brain. The catheter would perform two functions: provide ultrasound images of the tumor and increase the temperature at specific locations. The researchers hope doctors will be able to use the catheter along with chemotherapy drugs encased in liposomes. The catheter would melt the liposome shells and deliver the chemotherapy directly to the tumor, without damaging surrounding tissue. Experiments with animal models have suggested that creating such a catheter for use in humans is possible.

chemotherapy. Specific drugs are being developed to protect organs such as the heart, kidneys, and bladder.

In addition, researchers are attempting to develop a new type of drug that would make radiation therapy more effective. This type of drug is called a radiosensitizer because it makes cancer cells more sensitive to radiation. However, this work is still in the early phases. It is unclear yet whether the radiosensitizers currently under investigation, such as misonidazole and metronidazole, will have the desired effect of making tumors more vulnerable to radiation.

10 GREAT QUESTIONS
TO ASK A DOCTOR

1. What type of brain tumor do I have, and where is it located?

2. What treatment do you recommend, and what are the goals of this treatment?

3. What are the risks and side effects of the treatment?

4. Are there other options besides this treatment?

5. What are the signs that the cancer might be getting worse? What are the signs that it is improving?

6. Are there medications I can take that would help with my symptoms?

7. What activities are OK for me to engage in?

8. What should I do if I experience problems in school?

9. Are there support groups that I can join for this illness?

10. Would seeing a physical or occupational therapist help me to overcome disabilities caused by the brain tumor?

Gene Therapy

Gene therapy is another
area being explored to
treat brain cancer. In gene
therapy, a specially designed
gene is inserted into deacti-
vated virus cells. These cells
are infused into the patient's
bloodstream. The virus par-
ticles enter the cancer cells
and insert the gene they carry
into the cancer cell's DNA.
When the cancer cells repro-
duce, the new cells incor-

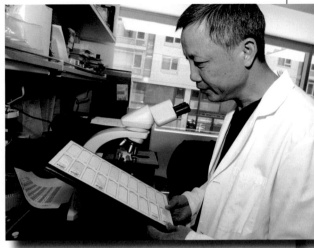

King Chiu, a researcher at the University
of California-San Francisco, examines
brain tumor samples. Cancer researchers
hope to translate new knowledge into
better treatments.

porate the implanted DNA. This new DNA inhibits (blocks) the
expression of the cancer-causing gene, replaces the defective gene
with a healthy gene, or initiates the production of a substance that
causes the defective cell to behave in a noncancerous way. Before
this method can be widely adopted, scientists must establish not
only that it will be effective but also that introducing a new gene
will not have unexpected consequences.

Immunotherapy

Immunotherapy approaches aim to use the patient's own immune
system to kill cancer cells. In one approach, the patient is given a

stimulant, such as interleukin-2, which is designed to enhance the patient's immune system activity. The idea is that the patient's own immune system cells will find and kill cancer cells. If the immune system's activity can be increased, then more cancer cells will be destroyed. Exactly how effective this type of approach will be is not yet clear.

Another immunotherapy approach that is being studied uses lab-grown antibodies to kill cancer cells. One such antibody is called a monoclonal antibody. "Monoclonal" means that the antibodies are all identical. This type of antibody is engineered to attach itself to cancer cells. Doctors attach a radioactive substance to these antibodies and inject them into the patient's body. The antibodies attach to the tumor, inserting the radiation into the cancer cells, killing them. This approach has shown some promise in treating certain types of cancer. However, it is not yet clear whether this approach will be successful in treating solid tumors such as those commonly found in brain cancer.

Researchers are very interested in the possibilities the immune system presents for using the body's own defenses against cancer. Cutting-edge studies in this area, together with research in the areas of chemotherapy, radiation therapy, and gene therapy, may help defeat one of humanity's most dreaded diseases. Someday, this research may lead to medical breakthroughs that will help dramatically swell the ranks of people who survive brain tumors and thrive many years after successful treatment.

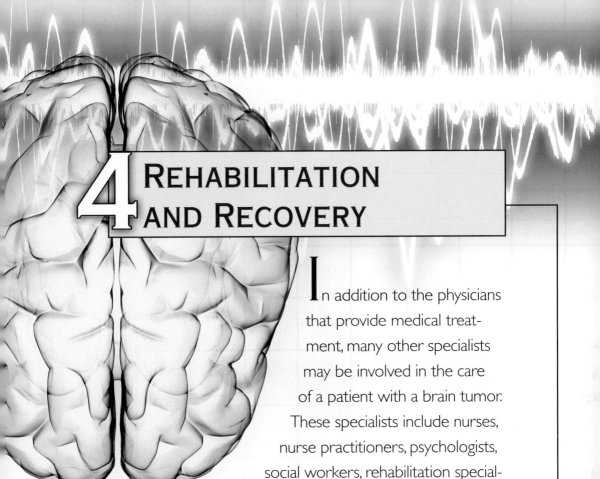

4 REHABILITATION AND RECOVERY

In addition to the physicians that provide medical treatment, many other specialists may be involved in the care of a patient with a brain tumor. These specialists include nurses, nurse practitioners, psychologists, social workers, rehabilitation specialists, and others. These professionals help patients manage the short-term and long-term issues related to recovery from brain cancer. After treatment for brain cancer, a patient may experience problems as a result of the cancer and the side effects of treatments. Depending on where the cancer was located, speech, movement, hearing, vision, or cognitive functions may be affected.

If a patient has difficulties in any of these areas, he or she will be referred to one or more therapists for rehabilitation. This may involve working with specialists who treat particular problems.

Rehabilitation Specialties

Rehabilitation experts include physical, occupational, speech, cognitive rehabilitation, and vision therapists. Cognitive rehabilitation therapists help patients relearn cognitive skills that have been affected by the cancer or cancer treatment. Physical therapists work with patients to improve movement and physical functioning. Occupational therapists help patients develop techniques to compensate for disabilities in their home and work environments. Speech therapists work with patients to improve their ability to speak. Vision therapists deal with patients' sight problems.

Cognitive and Psychological Rehabilitation

If you experience problems with thinking, memory, or other mental and personality-related problems, these issues can be addressed with cognitive rehabilitation. You may work with a cognitive rehabilitation therapist, who will teach you techniques for dealing with deficits such as memory loss.

Brain cancer sometimes affects areas of the brain that control emotions or self-control. This can result in sudden mood swings or inappropriate behavior. Psychotherapists provide assistance with dealing with emotional problems—those that result from damage to the areas of the brain that affect emotion, and those relating to the traumatic experience of cancer diagnosis and treatment. Psychotherapists also play a key role

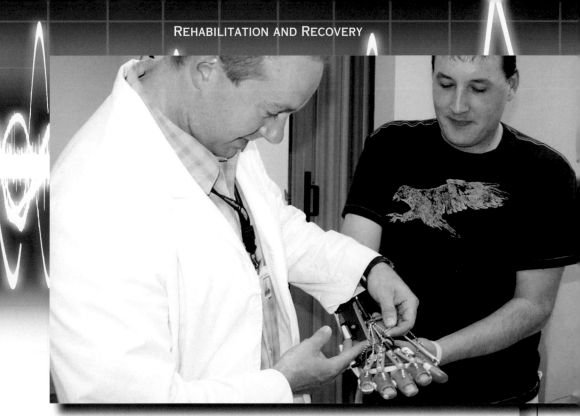

An occupational therapy assistant (left) adjusts the SaeboFlex on Mark Chrudimsky (right), who had surgery for a brain tumor. The device's spring system supports the weakened wrist and hand and helps the patient open and close the fingers.

at the beginning of rehabilitation by administering a standard set of tests for cognitive and emotional functioning. Other therapists can use the results of these tests as a road map for administering appropriate therapy.

Physical and Occupational Therapy

It is not uncommon for someone with a brain tumor to have some physical effects after treatment. Common problems are weakness in one or more limbs, difficulty with balance, and

47

tremors (shaking). If you experience such physical problems, a physical therapist can provide exercises and other treatments designed to help you improve your physical abilities. For example, treatments may focus on strengthening weakened parts of the body or improving your balance and ability to walk.

Occupational therapy is a form of therapy that helps individuals achieve independence in their everyday lives. An occupational therapist can help you identify skills affected by your brain tumor, such as taking a shower and getting dressed, and come up with ways to help you accomplish your tasks. The therapist can help you improve your skills by practicing specific exercises and activities. If necessary, the therapist can teach you to perform activities in a different way or to use assistive equipment.

Speech and Vision Therapy

If your speech is affected, a speech therapist can provide exercises to help you regain or improve your ability to speak. He or she can also teach you alternative ways of communicating if necessary. Speech therapists can also help patients deal with difficulties related to swallowing food.

Some types of tumors affect a person's sight. This can happen when a tumor affects the visual cortex (the part of the brain responsible for processing sight) or when the tumor is located on the optic nerve, which runs from the back of the eye to the brain. If you experience a full or partial loss of sight, a therapist can provide training in techniques that you can use to get around and function in the world. Following brain cancer, you may retain some vision but have trouble seeing. In this case, a vision therapist can provide training in using devices such as special monitors that magnify book or news-paper pages.

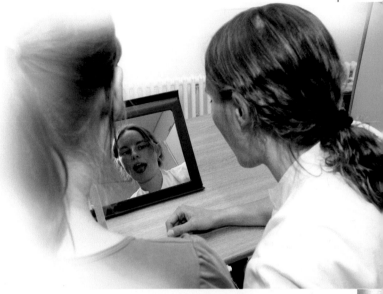

A speech therapist teaches a patient exercises to improve her ability to speak clearly. Speech therapists help patients who have had damage to the speech center of the brain.

Returning to School

A student may feel frustrated by the limitations resulting from brain cancer when returning to school. If you experience physical issues with movement, hearing, or sight, then you may feel self-conscious and embarrassed. All of this can be very stressful, and the stress itself can make the situation worse. Be aware that there are special devices that you can use to assist you with seeing and hearing better in class. The rehabilitation

Growth Issues

Depending on the age when you develop brain cancer, you may or may not have reached your full growth. If the cancer occurs in the region of the pituitary gland, which produces hormones that regulate growth, then these hormones may no longer be produced after treatment. This could prevent you from growing to a normal height. Therefore, it is important for your growth to be monitored. If you are a young teenager and do not appear to be growing normally, it may be necessary to take injections of growth hormones to achieve normal growth.

therapists you will work with after your treatment can recommend devices that will be helpful in your case. They can also explain to you and your parents how to obtain them and how to use them.

It's important for you and your parents to involve your teachers and other school personnel in arranging for special assistance in your classes. It is especially important to make your teachers aware of your capabilities as well as your limitations. For example, if your sight or hearing is limited but you are otherwise quite capable of learning in a normal academic program, then it is important for your teachers to understand this.

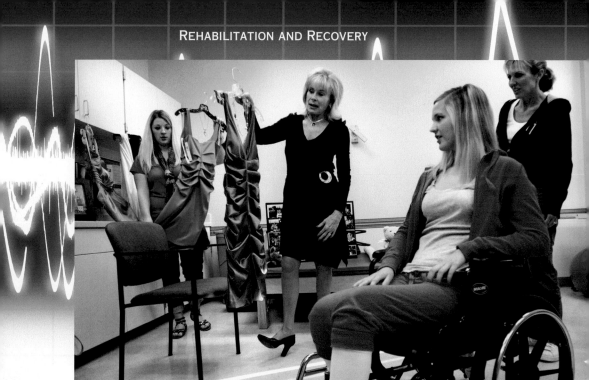

Brittany Claunch, a teen recovering from brain tumor surgery, looks at prom dresses with the help of representatives from Nordstrom. While the tumor paralyzed part of her body, Claunch was well enough to attend her 2009 junior prom.

People are often uncomfortable with things they are unfamiliar with or that are different from their usual experience. Therefore, it is possible that some of your classmates may avoid you or tease you. If you encounter difficulties with other students, be sure to tell your parents and teachers about such problems so that they can deal with them. Don't assume, however, that your experiences with other students will necessarily be negative. Fellow classmates often turn out to be surprisingly helpful, supportive, and sympathetic, especially in a crisis or its aftermath.

Coping with Life Changes

There are a number of things that you can do to help your-self overcome obstacles on the road to recovery. The first is to take care of yourself physically. Eat a healthy, well-balanced diet and get adequate rest and exercise. This will help you stay in the best possible condition to cope with the physical demands and stresses of treatment and recovery.

It is best to consider in advance the changes you may experience. If you don't know what to expect, ask questions of all the doctors and therapists you encounter. Then, prepare a strategy for coping with potential limitations. Be aware that not all side effects are permanent. Some conditions improve over time. As you go back to school and other activities, you may wish to work with a counselor or psychotherapist with whom you can discuss any anger or frustration you may experience.

It is very important to have support when coping with the effects of a brain tumor. There are many support groups for both patients and their families. These groups can pro-vide vital emotional support and social interaction as well as practical advice. Information on local support groups, including meeting places and meeting times, can be found in local newspapers and through local hospitals or health centers.

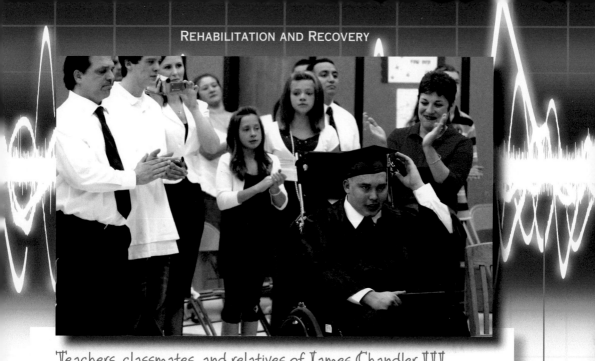

Teachers, classmates, and relatives of James Chandler III applaud as he receives his high school diploma in Antioch, California. Chandler successfully graduated in 2007 before passing away from an inoperable brain tumor in 2008.

There are many things that you cannot control when you have a disease like brain cancer. However, it is important to focus on the areas in which you do have influence. You can develop coping strategies and participate in making decisions. This fosters a sense of control and can help you deal with challenges.

It is not easy to cope with all the life changes that a brain tumor may bring. However, it is important to stay involved with friends, school, and other community activities as much as you can. Despite any limitations that you may encounter, remaining active and involved will allow you to continue to grow as a person and maintain a positive outlook as you recover from this illness.

Glossary

benign tumor A slow-growing tumor that is unlikely to metastasize.

cerebellum The part of the brain above and behind the brain stem. The cerebellum controls bodily balance and other complex motor functions.

cerebrum The front and upper part of the brain that consists of two hemispheres and connecting structures. The cerebrum is believed to control voluntary movement and higher mental functions, such as thought, reason, memory, and emotion.

chemotherapy The use of chemical agents in the treatment or control of a disease, such as cancer.

cognitive Relating to mental activities, such as thinking, reasoning, remembering, and using language.

convulsions Involuntary contractions of the muscles that shake the body violently.

craniotomy Surgical opening of the skull.

gene A tiny part of DNA or RNA that controls the production of a specific protein that regulates a body function or trait or controls the activity of another gene or genes.

glial tumor A tumor that grows from the cells of the fibers that support the nerve cells in the brain; glioma.

malignant tumor A tumor that is fast-growing, is likely to spread, and is resistant to treatment.

metastasize To transmit cancerous cells from an original site to one or more sites elsewhere in the body.

myelin A fatty material that sheaths and protects the axons of the nerve cells of the brain and spinal cord.

neurologist A doctor who specializes in treating diseases of the brain and spinal cord.

nonglial tumor A tumor that grows from the cells of nerves, glands, or blood vessels in the brain.

occupational therapist An expert who helps people with disabilities develop techniques to meet the demands of daily living and work.

oncologist A doctor who specializes in treating cancer.

pituitary gland A gland in the brain that puts out hormones that regulate growth, among other things.

tumor A mass of cells that are reproducing and growing out of control.

For More Information

American Brain Tumor Association

2720 River Road

Des Plaines, IL 60018

(800) 886-2282

Web site: http://www.abta.org

The American Brain Tumor Association is a not-for-profit, independent organization. It seeks to eliminate brain tumors through research and meet the needs of brain tumor patients and their families.

American Cancer Society

250 Williams Street NW

Atlanta, GA 30303-1002

(800) 227-2345

Web site: http://www.cancer.org

The American Cancer Society is a nationwide, community-based, voluntary health organization dedicated to eliminating cancer as a major health problem. The organization works to prevent cancer, save lives, and diminish suffering through research, education, advocacy, and service.

Canadian Cancer Society

55 St. Clair Avenue West, Suite 300

Toronto, ON M4V 2Y7

Canada

(416) 961-7223

Web site: http://www.cancer.ca

The Canadian Cancer Society is a national, community-based organization of volunteers, whose mission is the eradication of cancer and the enhancement of the quality of life of people living with cancer.

Cancer Care Ontario

620 University Avenue

Toronto, ON M5G 2L7

Canada

(416) 971-9800

Web site: http://www.cancercare.on.ca

Cancer Care Ontario works to reduce the number of people diagnosed with cancer and make sure patients receive better care every step of the way.

Centers for Disease Control and Prevention (CDC)

1600 Clifton Road

Atlanta, GA 30333

(800) CDC-INFO [232-4636]

Web site: http://www.cdc.gov

The CDC, an operating component of the Department of Health and Human Services, is at the forefront of public health efforts to prevent and control infectious and chronic diseases, injuries, workplace hazards, disabilities, and environmental health threats.

Children's Brain Tumor Foundation

274 Madison Avenue, Suite 1004

New York, NY 10016

(866) CBT-HOPE [228-4673]

Web site: http://www.cbtf.org

This organization's mission is to improve the treatment, quality of life, and long-term outlook for children with brain and spinal cord tumors.

Mayo Clinic

200 First Street SW

Rochester, MN 55905

(507) 284-2511

Web site: http://www.mayoclinic.org

Mayo Clinic is a nonprofit worldwide leader in medical care, research, and education. Its staff members, including doctors, specialists, and other health care professionals, provide comprehensive diagnosis, understandable answers, and effective treatment.

National Brain Tumor Society

124 Watertown Street, Suite 2D

Watertown, MA 02472

(800) 770-8287

Web site: http://www.braintumor.org

The National Brain Tumor Society exists to find a cure for brain tumors and improve the quality of life of those affected by brain tumors. The organization invests in research and offers education, information, and caring support to patients, families, and caregivers.

National Cancer Institute (NCI)

Public Inquiries Office

6116 Executive Boulevard, Suite 300

Bethesda, MD 20892-8322

(800) 4-CANCER [422-6237]

Web site: http://www.cancer.gov

The NCI, a component of the National Institutes of Health, is the U.S. gov-
ernment's principal agency for cancer research and training. It coordinates
the National Cancer Program, which conducts and supports research,
training, health information dissemination, and other programs.

National Institute of Neurological Disorders and Stroke (NINDS)

P.O. Box 5801

Bethesda, MD 20824

(800) 352-9424

Web site: http://www.ninds.nih.gov

The mission of NINDS is to reduce the burden of neurological disease by
conducting, fostering, coordinating, and guiding research on the causes, prevention, diagnosis, and treatment of neurological disorders and stroke.

Web Sites

Due to the changing nature of Internet links, Rosen Publishing
has developed an online list of Web sites related to the subject
of this book. This site is updated regularly. Please use this link to
access the list:

http://www.rosenlinks.com/bdis/btum

For Further Reading

Bakewell, Lisa, and Karen Bellenir. *Cancer Information for Teens: Health Tips About Cancer Awareness, Prevention, Diagnosis, and Treatment* (Teen Health). 2nd ed. Detroit, MI: Omnigraphics, 2010.

Bingham, Jane. *Surviving Cancer* (Real Life Heroes). Mankato, MN: Arcturus Publishing, 2011.

Black, Peter McLaren. *Living with a Brain Tumor: Dr. Peter Black's Guide to Taking Control of Your Treatment.* New York, NY: Henry Holt, 2006.

Clark, Arda Darakjian. *Brain Tumors* (Diseases and Disorders). Detroit, MI: Thomson, Gale, 2006.

Dreyer, ZoAnn. *Living with Cancer* (Teen's Guides). New York, NY: Facts On File, 2008.

Dryburgh, Nicole. *The Way I See It.* London, England: Hodder Children's, 2008.

Feuerstein, Michael, and Patricia Findley. *The Cancer Survivor's Guide: The Essential Handbook to Life After Cancer.* New York, NY: Marlowe & Co., 2006.

Katz, Robert A. *Elaine's Circle: A Teacher, a Student, a Classroom, and One Unforgettable Year.* New York, NY: Avalon, 2005.

McGowan, Anthony. *Jack Tumor.* New York, NY: Farrar, Straus, and Giroux, 2009.

Parks, Peggy J. *Brain Tumors* (Compact Research). San Diego, CA: ReferencePoint Press, 2011.

Silverstein, Alvin, Virginia B. Silverstein, and Laura Silverstein Nunn. *Cancer* (Twenty-First Century Medical Library). Minneapolis, MN: Twenty-First Century Books, 2006.

Stark-Vance, Virginia, and M. L. Dubay. *100 Questions and Answers About Brain Tumors*. Boston, MA: Jones & Bartlett Publishers, 2004.

Stewart, Sheila, and Ida Walker. *Youth with Cancer: Facing the Shadows* (Helping Youth with Mental, Physical, and Social Challenges). Philadelphia, PA: Mason Crest Publishers, 2008.

Index

About the Authors

Louis J. Cook is an author with a special interest in health and science topics.

Jeri Freedman has a bachelor of arts degree from Harvard University. She is the author of more than thirty young adult nonfiction books, including books on various types of cancer, hemophilia, autism, and hepatitis B.

Photo Credits

Cover © www.istockphoto.com/Sebastian Kaulitzki; p. 8 © Kallista Images/CMSP; p. 10 © Dr. Cecil H. Fox/Photo Researchers, Inc.; p. 13 Dan McCoy/Rainbow/Science Faction/Getty Images; p. 16 Arctic-Images/The Image Bank/Getty Images; p. 20 © Henning Dalhoff/Bonnier Publications/Photo Researchers, Inc.; p. 22 © www.istockphoto.com/Joshua Blake; p. 24 iStockphoto/Thinkstock.com; p. 26 AbleStock.com/Thinkstock.com; p. 29 Dr. Giovanni Di Chiro/NCI; p. 33 © The Sacramento Bee/ZUMA Press; p. 35 Mark Harmel/Stone/Getty Images; p. 37 Steve Nagy/Design Pics/Getty Images; pp. 39, 47 © AP Images; p. 43 © Sean Donnelly/ZUMA Press; p. 49 © imagebroker.net/SuperStock; p. 51 © Sacramento Bee/ZUMA Press; p. 53 © Eddie Ledesma/Contra Costa Times/ZUMA Press; cover, back cover, and interior background images and elements (nerve cells, brain waves, brains) Shutterstock.com.

Designer: Les Kanturek; Editor: Andrea Sclarow; Photo Researcher: Amy Feinberg